Mediter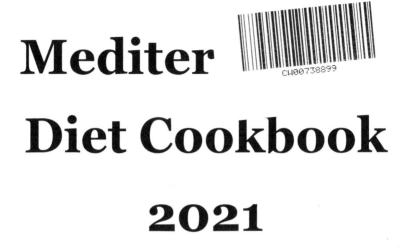

Diet Cookbook

2021

50 Affordable
Mediterranean Recipes

By Allison Bishop

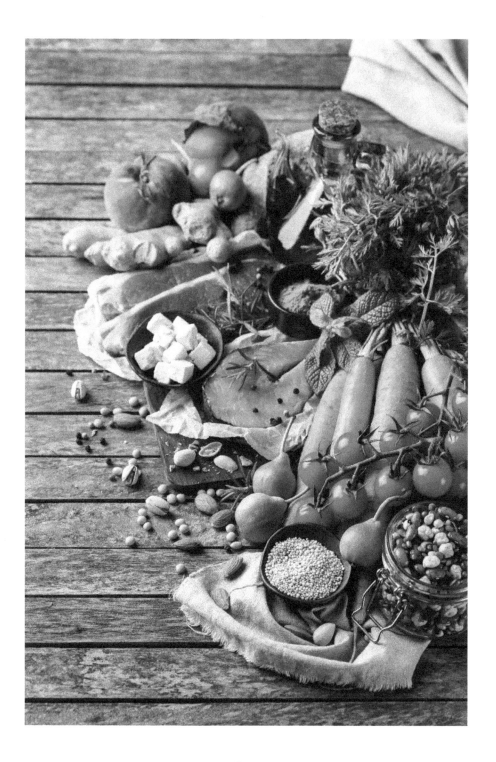

Table of Contents

Introduction

Mediterranean diet is based on the eating habits of the inhabitants of the regions along the Mediterranean Sea, mostly from Italy, Spain and Greece; it is considered more a life style then a diet, in fact it also promotes physical activity and proper liquid (mostly water) consumption.

Depending on fresh seasonal local foods there are no strict rules, because of the many cultural differences, but there are some common factors.

Mediterranean diet has become famous for its ability to reduce heart disease and obesity, thanks to the low consumption of unhealthy fats that increase blood glucose.

Mediterranean diet is mostly plant based, so it's rich of antioxidants; vegetables, fruits like apple and grapes, olive oil, whole grains, herbs, beans and nuts are consumed in large quantities.

Moderate amounts of poultry, eggs, dairy and seafood are also common aliments, accompanied by a little bit of red wine (some studies say that in small amount it helps to stay healthy).

Red meat and sweets like cookies and cakes are accepted but are more limited in quantity.

Foods to avoid:

- refined grains, such as white bread and pasta
- dough containing white flour refined oils (even canola oil and soybean oil)
- foods with added sugars (like pastries, sodas, and candies)

processed meats processed or packaged foods

Chapter 1: Breakfast and Snack Recipes

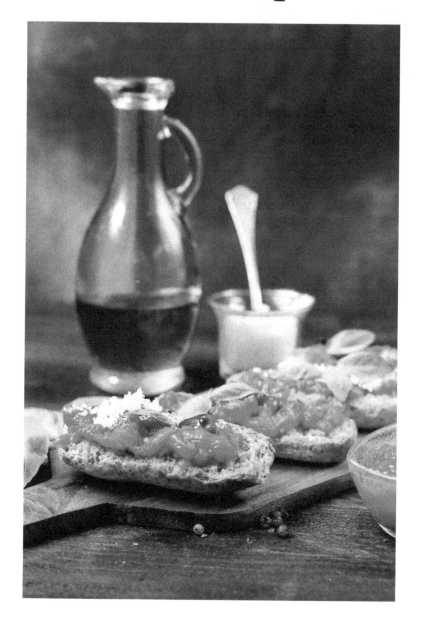

Olives And Cheese Stuffed Tomatoes

Servings: 24 | Cooking: 0 min

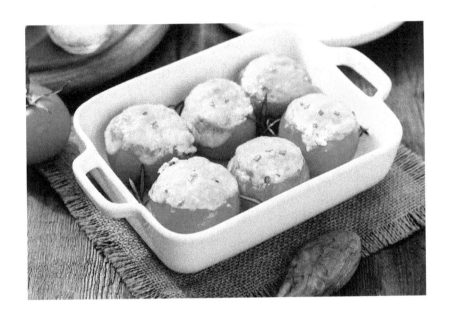

Ingredients

- 24 cherry tomatoes, top cut off and insides scooped out
- 2 tablespoons olive oil
- ¼ teaspoon red pepper flakes
- ½ cup feta cheese, crumbled
- 2 tablespoons black olive paste
- ¼ cup mint, torn

Directions

1. In a bowl, mix the olives paste with the rest of the ingredients except the cherry tomatoes and whisk well.
2. Stuff the cherry tomatoes with this mix, arrange them all on a platter and serve as an appetizer.

Nutrition: calories 136; fat 8.6; fiber 4.8; carbs 5.6; protein 5.1

Feta Cheese Log With Sun-dried Tomatoes And Kalamata Olives

Servings: 2 | Cooking: 20 min

Ingredients

- 8 ounces feta cheese, crumbled
- 4 ounces cream cheese, softened
- 2 tablespoons extra-virgin olive oil
- 1/8-1/4 teaspoon cayenne pepper (depending on your taste)
- 1/4 cup chopped sun-dried tomato
- 1/4 cup chopped Kalamata olive
- 1/2 teaspoon dried Mediterranean oregano, crumbled
- 1 small garlic clove, minced
- 1/2 cup walnuts, toasted, chopped
- 1/4 cup fresh parsley, minced

Directions

1. With a mixer, combine the feta cheese, cream cheese, and the olive oil on medium speed until

well combined. Add the remaining ingredients and mix well.

2. Shape the soft mixture into a 10-inch long log.

3. Combine the parsley and the walnuts; roll the log over the mixture, pressing slightly to stick the parsley and the walnuts on the sides of the log.

4. Wrap the log with plastic wrap; refrigerate for at least 5 hours to let the flavors blend.

5. Remove the plastic wrap, lay the log on a parsley-lined serving platter. Serve with whole-wheat crackers and toasted whole-wheat slices of baguette.

Nutrition:1154 cal., 106.3 g total fat (43.9 sat. fat), 226.2 mg chol., 2395.3 mg sodium, 23 g total carbs., 5 g fiber, 13.5 g sugar, and 35.2 g protein.

Lemon Salmon Rolls

Servings: 6 | Cooking: 0 min

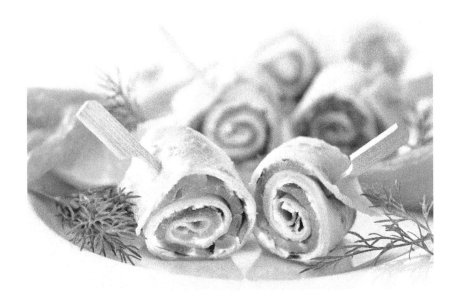

Ingredients

- 6 wonton wrappers
- 7 oz salmon, grilled
- 6 lettuce leaves
- 1 carrot, peeled
- 1 cucumber, trimmed
- 1 tablespoon lemon juice
- 1 teaspoon olive oil
- ¼ teaspoon dried oregano

Directions

1. Cut the carrot and cucumber onto the wedges.
2. Then chop the grilled salmon.
3. Arrange the salmon, carrot and cucumber wedges, and lettuce leaves on 6 wonton wraps.
4. In the shallow bowl whisk together dried oregano, olive oil, and lemon juice.
5. Sprinkle the roll mixture with oil dressing and wrap.

Nutrition: calories 90; fat 3.4; fiber 0.7; carbs 7.7; protein 7.7

Ginger And Cream Cheese Dip

Servings: 6 | Cooking: 0 min

Ingredients

- ½ cup ginger, grated
- 2 bunches cilantro, chopped
- 3 tablespoons balsamic vinegar
- ½ cup olive oil
- 1 and ½ cups cream cheese, soft

Directions

1. In your blender, mix the ginger with the rest of the ingredients and pulse well.
2. Divide into small bowls and serve as a party dip.

Nutrition: calories 213; fat 4.9; fiber 4.1; carbs 8.8; protein 17.8

Lemon Endive Bites

Servings: 10 | Cooking: 0 min

Ingredients

- 6 oz endive
- 2 pears, chopped
- 4 oz Blue cheese, crumbled
- 1 teaspoon olive oil
- 1 teaspoon lemon juice
- ¾ teaspoon ground cinnamon

Directions

1. Separate endive into the spears (10 spears).
2. In the bowl combine together chopped pears, olive oil, lemon juice, ground cinnamon, and Blue cheese.
3. Fill the endive spears with cheese mixture.

Nutrition: calories 72; fat 3.8; fiber 1.9; carbs 7.4; protein 2.8

Perfect Italian Potatoes

Servings: 6 | Cooking: 7 min

Ingredients

- 2 lbs baby potatoes, clean and cut in half
- 3/4 cup vegetable broth
- 6 oz Italian dry dressing mix

Directions

1. Add all ingredients into the inner pot of instant pot and stir well.
2. Seal pot with lid and cook on high for 7 minutes.
3. Once done, allow to release pressure naturally for 3 minutes then release remaining using quick release. Remove lid.
4. Stir well and serve.

Nutrition: Calories 149 Fat 0.3 g Carbohydrates 41.6 g Sugar 11.4 g Protein 4.5 g Cholesterol 0 mg

Feta Artichoke Dip

Servings: 8 | Cooking: 30 min

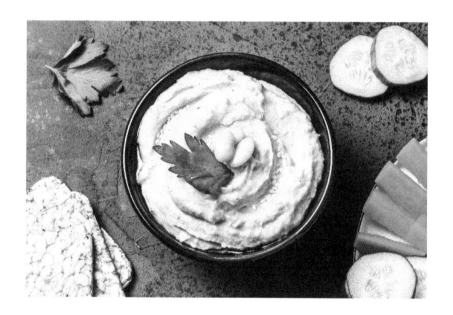

Ingredients

- 8 ounces artichoke hearts, drained and quartered
- ¾ cup basil, chopped
- ¾ cup green olives, pitted and chopped
- 1 cup parmesan cheese, grated
- 5 ounces feta cheese, crumbled

Directions

1. In your food processor, mix the artichokes with the basil and the rest of the ingredients, pulse well, and transfer to a baking dish.
2. Introduce in the oven, bake at 375 degrees F for 30 minutes and serve as a party dip.

Nutrition: calories 186; fat 12.4; fiber 0.9; carbs 2.6; protein 1.5

Peach Skewers

Servings: 2 | Cooking: 0 min

Ingredients

- 1 peach
- 4 Mozzarella balls, cherry size
- ½ teaspoon pistachio, chopped
- 1 teaspoon honey

Directions

1. Cut the peach on 4 cubes.
2. Then skewer peach cubes and Mozzarella balls on the skewers.
3. Sprinkle them with honey and chopped pistachio.

Nutrition: calories 202; fat 14.3; fiber 1.2; carbs 10; protein 10.8

Chickpeas Salsa

Servings: 6 | Cooking: 0 min

Ingredients

- 4 spring onions, chopped
- 1 cup baby spinach
- 15 ounces canned chickpeas, drained and rinsed
- Salt and black pepper to the taste
- 2 tablespoons olive oil
- 2 tablespoons lemon juice
- 1 tablespoon cilantro, chopped

Directions

1. In a bowl, mix the chickpeas with the spinach, spring onions and the rest of the ingredients, toss, divide into small cups and serve as a snack.

Nutrition: calories 224; fat 5.1; fiber 1; carbs 9.9; protein 15.1

Hummus Appetizer Bites

Servings: 1 Bite | Cooking: 10 min

Ingredients

- 11/4 cups all-purpose flour
- 1/2 tsp. salt
- 5 TB. cold butter
- 2 TB. vegetable shortening
- 1/4 cup ice water
- 1 batch Traditional Hummus (recipe in Chapter 11)
- 1 tsp. paprika
- 12 kalamata olives
- 12 fresh parsley leaves

Directions

1. In a food processor fitted with a chopping blade, pulse 1 cup all-purpose flour and salt 5 times.
2. Add cold butter and vegetable shortening, and pulse for 1 minute or until mixture resembles coarse meal.
3. Continue to pulse while adding water for about 1 minute. Test dough; if it holds together when you

pinch it, it doesn't require any additional moisture. If it does not come together, add another 3 tablespoons water.

4. Remove dough from the food processor, place in a plastic bag, form into a flat disc, and refrigerate for 30 minutes.

5. Preheat the oven to 425°F.

6. Remove dough from the plastic bag, and dust both sides with flour. Sprinkle your counter with flour.

7. Using a rolling pin, roll out dough to 1/4 inch thickness. Using a 2-inch circle cookie cutter, cut out 12 circles of dough. Gently mold dough circles into a mini muffin tin, and using a fork, gently poke dough.

8. Bake for 10 minutes. Remove from the oven, and set aside to cool.

9. Spoon about 1 tablespoon Traditional Hummus on top of each cooled piecrust, sprinkle with paprika, and top with 1 kalamata olive and 1 parsley leaf each. Serve immediately or refrigerate.

Chapter 2: Lunch & Dinner Recipes

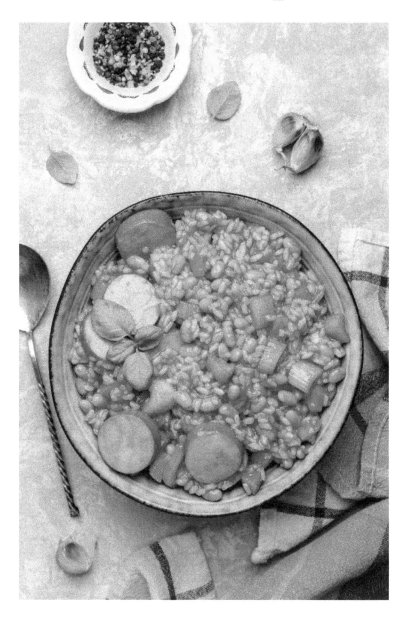

Carrot And Potato Soup

Servings: 6 | Cooking: 35 min

Ingredients

- 5 cups beef broth
- 4 carrots, peeled
- 1 teaspoon dried thyme
- ½ teaspoon ground cumin
- 1 teaspoon salt
- 1 ½ cup potatoes, chopped
- 1 tablespoon olive oil
- ½ teaspoon ground black pepper
- 1 tablespoon lemon juice
- 1/3 cup fresh parsley, chopped
- 1 chili pepper, chopped
- 1 tablespoon tomato paste
- 1 tablespoon sour cream

Directions

1. Line the baking tray with baking paper.
2. Put sweet potatoes and carrot on the tray and sprinkle with olive oil and salt.

3. Bake the vegetables for 25 minutes at 365F.
4. Meanwhile, pour the beef broth in the pan and bring it to boil.
5. Add dried thyme, ground cumin, chopped chili pepper, and tomato paste.
6. When the vegetables are cooked, add them in the pan.
7. Boil the vegetables until they are soft.
8. Then blend the mixture with the help of the blender until smooth.
9. Simmer it for 2 minutes and add lemon juice. Stir well.
10. Then add sour cream and chopped parsley. Stir well.
11. Simmer the soup for 3 minutes more.

Nutrition: calories 123; fat 4.1; fiber 2.9; carbs 16.4; protein 5.3

Macedonian Greens And Cheese Pie

Servings: 6 | Cooking: 50 min

Ingredients

- 1 bunch chicory
- 1 bunch rocket or arugula
- 1 bunch mint
- 1 bunch dill
- 10 sheets whole-wheat filo pastry
- 150 g halloumi, finely diced
- 150 g ricotta
- 200 g baby spinach
- 250 g Greek feta, crumbled
- 4 eggs
- 50 g dried whole-wheat breadcrumbs
- 6 green onions, trimmed
- Olive oil, to brush

Directions

1. Trim the rocket stalks and the chicory. Finely chop the green onions and the dill (include the dill stems). Strip the mint leaves.

2. Pour water into a large-sized pan; bring to boil. Ready a bowl with iced water beside the stove. Add the chicory into the boiling water; blanch for 3 minutes and using a slotted spoon, transfer to the bowl with iced water. Repeat the process with the spinach and the rocket, blanching each for 1 minute; drain well.

3. A handful at a time, tightly wring the greens to squeeze out the excess liquid, then pat dry with paper towel. Finely chop the blanched greens. Combine them with the eggs, herbs, feta, 30 g of the breadcrumbs, ricotta, and 3/4 of the halloumi; season.

4. Preheat the oven to 180C.

5. Grease a 5-cm deep 25cmx pie tin.

6. Brush a filo sheet with the olive oil, place it in the pie tin, extending the edge of the filo outside the edge of the tin. Brush the remaining sheets of filo and add them to the pie tin, arranging them like wheel spokes.

7. Sprinkle the remaining breadcrumbs over the base of the layered filo sheets. Top with the filling mixture. Loosely fold the filo sheets over to cover

the filling, brush with oil, sprinkle with water, and scatter the halloumi over.

8. Bake for 45 minutes. After 45 minutes, cover, and bake for additional 15 minutes, or until heated through.

Nutrition:374.8 Cal, 20 g total fat (12 g sat. fat), 22 g carb., 2 g fiber, 3 g sugar, 25g protein, and 1506.7 mg sodium.

Chicken Stuffed Peppers

Servings: 6 | Cooking: 0 min

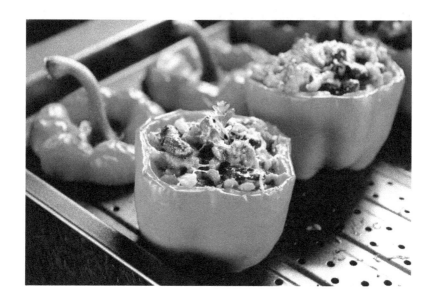

Ingredients

- 1 cup Greek yogurt
- 2 tablespoons mustard
- Salt and black pepper to the taste
- 1 pound rotisserie chicken meat, cubed
- 4 celery stalks, chopped
- 2 tablespoons balsamic vinegar
- 1 bunch scallions, sliced
- ¼ cup parsley, chopped

- 1 cucumber, sliced
- 3 red bell peppers, halved and deseeded
- 1 pint cherry tomatoes, quartered

Directions

1. In a bowl, mix the chicken with the celery and the rest of the ingredients except the bell peppers and toss well.
2. Stuff the peppers halves with the chicken mix and serve for lunch.

Nutrition: calories 266; fat 12.2; fiber 4.5; carbs 15.7; protein 3.7

Turkey Fritters And Sauce

Servings: 4 | Cooking: 30 min

Ingredients

- 2 garlic cloves, minced
- 1 egg
- 1 red onion, chopped
- 1 tablespoon olive oil
- ¼ teaspoon red pepper flakes
- 1 pound turkey meat, ground
- ½ teaspoon oregano, dried
- Cooking: spray
- For the sauce:
- 1 cup Greek yogurt
- 1 cucumber, chopped
- 1 tablespoon olive oil
- ¼ teaspoon garlic powder
- 2 tablespoons lemon juice
- ¼ cup parsley, chopped

Directions

1. Heat up a pan with 1 tablespoon oil over medium heat, add the onion and the garlic, sauté for 5 minutes, cool down and transfer to a bowl.
2. Add the meat, turkey, oregano and pepper flakes, stir and shape medium fritters out of this mix.
3. Heat up another pan greased with cooking spray over medium-high heat, add the turkey fritters and brown for 5 minutes on each side.
4. Introduce the pan in the oven and bake the fritters at 375 degrees F for 15 minutes more.
5. Meanwhile, in a bowl, mix the yogurt with the cucumber, oil, garlic powder, lemon juice and parsley and whisk really well.
6. Divide the fritters between plates, spread the sauce all over and serve for lunch.

Nutrition: calories 364; fat 16.8; fiber 5.5; carbs 26.8; protein 23.4

Garlic Clove Roasted Chicken

Servings: 8 | Cooking: 1 ½ Hours

Ingredients

- 8 chicken legs
- 40 garlic cloves, crushed
- 1 shallot, sliced
- ½ cup white wine
- 1 bay leaf
- 1 thyme sprig
- Salt and pepper to taste

Directions

1. Season the chicken with salt and pepper.
2. Combine it with the rest of the ingredients in a deep dish baking pan.
3. Cover the pan with aluminum foil and cook in the preheated oven at 350F for 1 hour.
4. Serve the chicken warm and fresh.

Nutrition: Calories:225 Fat:7.5g Protein:29.9g Carbohydrates:5.6g

Chapter 3: Meat Recipes

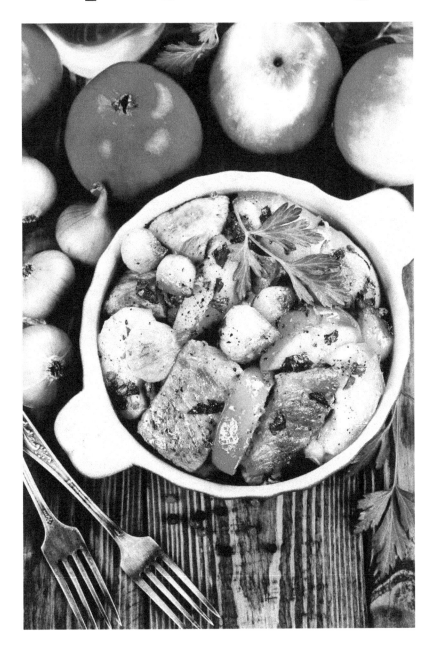

Chicken Quinoa Pilaf

Servings: 1 Cup | Cooking: 35 min

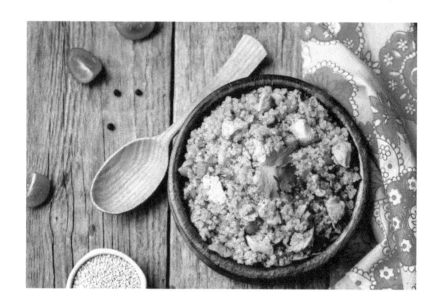

Ingredients

- 2 (8-oz.) boneless, skinless chicken breasts, cut into 1/2-in. cubes
- 3 TB. extra-virgin olive oil
- 1 medium red onion, finely chopped
- 1 TB. minced garlic
- 1 (16-oz.) can diced tomatoes, with juice
- 2 cups water
- 2 tsp. salt

- 1 TB. dried oregano
- 1 TB. turmeric
- 1 tsp. paprika
- 1 tsp. ground black pepper
- 2 cups red or yellow quinoa
- 1/2 cup fresh parsley, chopped

Directions

1. In a large, 3-quart pot over medium heat, heat extra-virgin olive oil. Add chicken, and cook for 5 minutes.
2. Add red onion and garlic, stir, and cook for 5 minutes.
3. Add tomatoes with juice, water, salt, oregano, turmeric, paprika, and black pepper. Stir, and simmer for 5 minutes.
4. Add red quinoa, and stir. Cover, reduce heat to low, and cook for 20 minutes. Remove from heat.
5. Fluff with a fork, cover again, and let sit for 10 minutes.
6. Serve warm.

Greek Styled Lamb Chops

Servings: 4 | Cooking: 4 min

Ingredients

- ¼ tsp black pepper
- ½ tsp salt
- 1 tbsp bottled minced garlic
- 1 tbsp dried oregano
- 2 tbsp lemon juice
- 8 pcs of lamb loin chops, around 4 oz
- Cooking: spray

Directions

1. Preheat broiler.
2. In a big bowl or dish, combine the black pepper, salt, minced garlic, lemon juice and oregano. Then rub it equally on all sides of the lamb chops.
3. Then coat a broiler pan with the cooking spray before placing the lamb chops on the pan and broiling until desired doneness is reached or for four minutes.

Nutrition: Calories: 131.9; Carbs: 2.6g; Protein: 17.1g; Fat: 5.9g

Bulgur And Chicken Skillet

Servings: 4 | Cooking: 40 min

Ingredients

- 4 (6-oz.) skinless, boneless chicken breasts
- 1 tablespoon olive oil, divided
- 1 cup thinly sliced red onion
- 1 tablespoon thinly sliced garlic
- 1 cup unsalted chicken stock
- 1 tablespoon coarsely chopped fresh dill
- 1/2 teaspoon freshly ground black pepper, divided
- 1/2 cup uncooked bulgur
- 2 teaspoons chopped fresh or 1/2 tsp. dried oregano
- 4 cups chopped fresh kale (about 2 1/2 oz.)
- 1/2 cup thinly sliced bottled roasted red bell peppers
- 2 ounces feta cheese, crumbled (about 1/2 cup)
- 3/4 teaspoon kosher salt, divided

Directions

1. Place a cast iron skillet on medium high fire and heat for 5 minutes. Add oil and heat for 2 minutes.

2. Season chicken with pepper and salt to taste.

3. Brown chicken for 4 minutes per side and transfer to a plate.

4. In same skillet, sauté garlic and onion for 3 minutes. Stir in oregano and bulgur and toast for 2 minutes.

5. Stir in kale and bell pepper, cook for 2 minutes. Pour in stock and season well with pepper and salt.

6. Return chicken to skillet and turn off fire. Pop in a preheated 400oF oven and bake for 15 minutes.

7. Remove form oven, fluff bulgur and turn over chicken. Let it stand for 5 minutes.

8. Serve and enjoy with a sprinkle of feta cheese.

Nutrition: Calories: 369; Carbs: 21.0g; Protein: 45.0g; Fats: 11.3g

Kibbeh With Yogurt

Servings: 1 Kibbeh | Cooking: 50 min

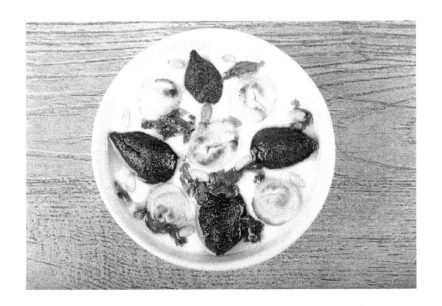

Ingredients

- 1/2 cup bulgur wheat, grind #1
- 4 cups water
- 1 large yellow onion, chopped
- 2 fresh basil leaves
- 1 lb. lean ground chuck beef
- 2 tsp. salt
- 1 tsp. ground black pepper
- 1/2 tsp. ground allspice

- 1/2 tsp. ground coriander
- 1/2 tsp. ground cumin
- 1/2 tsp. ground nutmeg
- 1/2 tsp. ground cloves
- 1/2 tsp. ground cinnamon
- 1/2 tsp. dried sage
- 1/4 cup long-grain rice
- 1/2 lb. ground beef
- 3 TB. extra-virgin olive oil
- 1/2 cup pine nuts
- 1 tsp. seven spices
- 4 cups Greek yogurt
- 2 TB. minced garlic
- 1 tsp. dried mint

Directions

1. In a small bowl, soak bulgur wheat in 1 cup water for 30 minutes.
2. In a food processor fitted with a chopping blade, blend 1/2 of yellow onion and basil for 30 seconds. Add bulgur, and blend for 30 more seconds.

3. Add ground chuck, 11/2 teaspoons salt, black pepper, allspice, coriander, cumin, nutmeg, cloves, cinnamon, and sage, and blend for 1 minute.
4. Transfer mixture to a large bowl, and knead for 3 minutes.
5. In a large pot, combine long-grain rice and remaining 3 cups water, and cook for 30 minutes.
6. In a medium skillet over medium heat, brown beef for 5 minutes, breaking up chunks with a wooden spoon.
7. Add remaining 1/2 of yellow onion, extra-virgin olive oil, remaining 1/2 teaspoon salt, pine nuts, and seven spices, and cook for 7 minutes. Set aside to cool.
8. Whisk Greek yogurt into cooked rice, add garlic and mint, reduce heat to low, and cook for 5 minutes.
9. Form meat-bulgur mixture into 12 equal-size balls. Create a groove in center of each ball, fill with beef and onion mixture, and seal groove.
10. Carefully drop balls into yogurt sauce, and cook for 15 minutes. Serve warm.

Mustard Chops With Apricot-basil Relish

Servings: 4 | Cooking: 12 min

Ingredients

- ¼ cup basil, finely shredded
- ¼ cup olive oil
- ½ cup mustard
- ¾ lb. fresh apricots, stone removed, and fruit diced
- 1 shallot, diced small
- 1 tsp ground cardamom
- 3 tbsp raspberry vinegar
- 4 pork chops
- Pepper and salt

Directions

1. Make sure that pork chops are defrosted well. Season with pepper and salt. Slather both sides of each pork chop with mustard. Preheat grill to medium-high fire.
2. In a medium bowl, mix cardamom, olive oil, vinegar, basil, shallot, and apricots. Toss to

combine and season with pepper and salt, mixing once again.

3. Grill chops for 5 to 6 minutes per side. As you flip, baste with mustard.

4. Serve pork chops with the Apricot-Basil relish and enjoy.

Nutrition: Calories: 486.5; Carbs: 7.3g; Protein: 42.1g; Fat: 32.1g

Chapter 4: Poultry Recipes

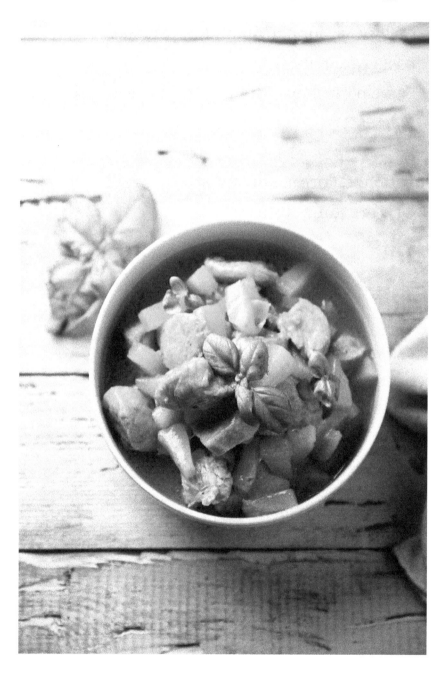

Chicken Kebabs

Servings: 4 | Cooking: 20 min

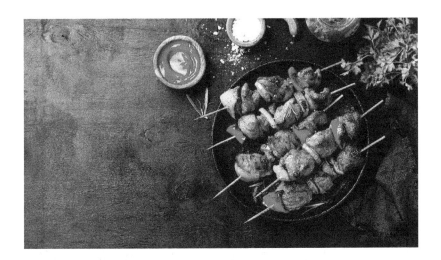

Ingredients

- 2 chicken breasts, skinless, boneless and cubed
- 1 red bell pepper, cut into squares
- 1 red onion, roughly cut into squares
- 2 teaspoons sweet paprika
- 1 teaspoon nutmeg, ground
- 1 teaspoon Italian seasoning
- ¼ teaspoon smoked paprika
- A pinch of salt and black pepper
- ¼ teaspoon cardamom, ground
- Juice of 1 lemon

- 3 garlic cloves, minced
- ½ cup olive oil

Directions

1. In a bowl, combine the chicken with the onion, the bell pepper and the other ingredients, toss well, cover the bowl and keep in the fridge for 30 minutes.
2. Assemble skewers with chicken, peppers and the onions, place them on your preheated grill and cook over medium heat for 8 minutes on each side.
3. Divide the kebabs between plates and serve with a side salad.

Nutrition: calories 262; fat 14; fiber 2; carbs 14; protein 20

Chicken, Corn And Peppers

Servings: 4 | Cooking: 1 Hour

Ingredients

- 2 pounds chicken breast, skinless, boneless and cubed
- 2 tablespoons olive oil
- 2 garlic cloves, minced
- 1 red onion, chopped
- 2 red bell peppers, chopped
- ¼ teaspoon cumin, ground
- 2 cups corn
- ½ cup chicken stock
- 1 teaspoon chili powder
- ¼ cup cilantro, chopped

Directions

1. Heat up a pot with the oil over medium-high heat, add the chicken and brown for 4 minutes on each side.
2. Add the onion and the garlic and sauté for 5 minutes more.

3. Add the rest of the ingredients, stir, bring to a simmer over medium heat and cook for 45 minutes.
4. Divide into bowls and serve.

Nutrition: calories 332; fat 16.1; fiber 8.4; carbs 25.4; protein 17.4

Spicy Cumin Chicken

Servings: 4 | Cooking: 25 min

Ingredients

- 2 teaspoons chili powder
- 2 and ½ tablespoons olive oil
- Salt and black pepper to the taste
- 1 and ½ teaspoons garlic powder
- 1 tablespoon smoked paprika
- ½ cup chicken stock
- 1 pound chicken breasts, skinless, boneless and halved
- 2 teaspoons sherry vinegar
- 2 teaspoons hot sauce
- 2 teaspoons cumin, ground
- ½ cup black olives, pitted and sliced

Directions

1. Heat up a pan with the oil over medium-high heat, add the chicken and brown for 3 minutes on each side.
2. Add the chili powder, salt, pepper, garlic powder and paprika, toss and cook for 4 minutes more.

3. Add the rest of the ingredients, toss, bring to a simmer and cook over medium heat for 15 minutes more.
4. Divide the mix between plates and serve.

Nutrition: calories 230; fat 18.4; fiber 9.4; carbs 15.3; protein 13.4

Chives Chicken And Radishes

Servings: 4 | Cooking: 30 min

Ingredients

- 2 chicken breasts, skinless, boneless and cubed
- Salt and black pepper to the taste
- 1 tablespoon olive oil
- 1 cup chicken stock
- ½ cup tomato sauce
- ½ pound red radishes, cubed
- 2 tablespoon chives, chopped

Directions

1. Heat up a Dutch oven with the oil over medium-high heat, add the chicken and brown for 4 minutes on each side.
2. Add the rest of the ingredients except the chives, bring to a simmer and cook over medium heat for 20 minutes.
3. Divide the mix between plates, sprinkle the chives on top and serve.

Nutrition: calories 277; fat 15; fiber 9.3; carbs 20.9; protein 33.2

Yogurt Chicken And Red Onion Mix

Servings: 4 | Cooking: 30 min

Ingredients

- 2 pounds chicken breast, skinless, boneless and sliced
- 3 tablespoons olive oil
- ¼ cup Greek yogurt
- 2 garlic cloves, minced
- ½ teaspoon onion powder
- A pinch of salt and black pepper
- 4 red onions, sliced

Directions

1. In a roasting pan, combine the chicken with the oil, the yogurt and the other ingredients, introduce in the oven at 375 degrees F and bake for 30 minutes.
2. Divide chicken mix between plates and serve hot.

Nutrition: calories 278; fat 15; fiber 9.2; carbs 15.1; protein 23.3

Basil Chicken With Olives

Servings: 5 | Cooking: 40 min

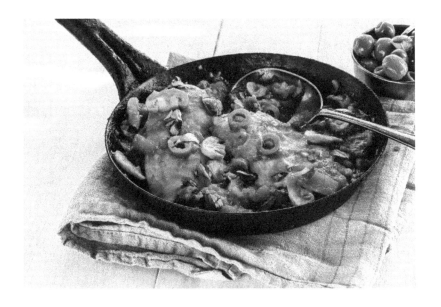

Ingredients

- 1.5-pound chicken breast, skinless, boneless
- 3 Kalamata olives, chopped
- 1 teaspoon minced garlic
- 1 teaspoon salt
- 1 teaspoon ground black pepper
- 2 tablespoons sunflower oil
- 1 tablespoon fresh basil, chopped
- ½ teaspoon chili flakes

- 1 tablespoon lemon juice
- ½ teaspoon honey
- ¼ cup of water

Directions

1. Combine together Kalamata olives, minced garlic, salt, ground black pepper, sunflower oil, basil, chili flakes, lemon juice, and honey.
2. Whisk the mixture until homogenous.
3. Chop the chicken breast roughly and arrange it in the baking dish.
4. Pour olives mixture over the chicken.
5. Then mix up it with the help of the fingertips.
6. Add water and cover the baking dish with foil.
7. Pierce the foil with the help of the fork or knife to give the "air" for meat during cooking.
8. Bake the chicken for 40 minutes at 360F.

Nutrition: calories 213; fat 9.3; fiber 0.2; carbs 1.3; protein 29

Chapter 5: Fish and Seafood Recipes

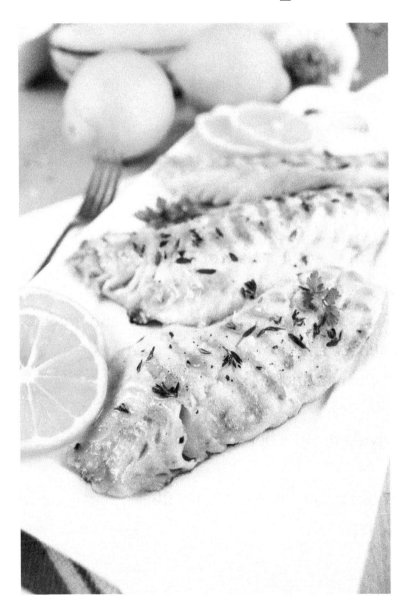

Cod And Cabbage

Servings: 4 | Cooking: 15 min

Ingredients

- 3 cups green cabbage, shredded
- 1 sweet onion, sliced
- A pinch of salt and black pepper
- ½ cup feta cheese, crumbled
- 4 teaspoons olive oil
- 4 cod fillets, boneless
- ¼ cup green olives, pitted and chopped

Directions

1. Grease a roasting pan with the oil, add the fish, the cabbage and the rest of the ingredients, introduce in the pan and cook at 450 degrees F for 15 minutes.
2. Divide the mix between plates and serve.

Nutrition: calories 270; fat 10; fiber 3; carbs 12; protein 31

Pecan Salmon Fillets

Servings: 6 | Cooking: 15 min

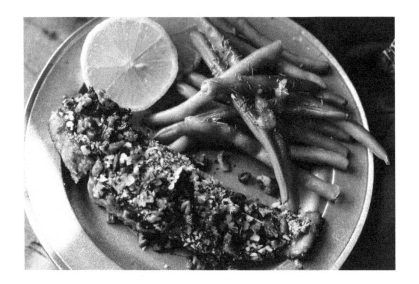

Ingredients

- 3 tablespoons olive oil
- 3 tablespoons mustard
- 5 teaspoons honey
- 1 cup pecans, chopped
- 6 salmon fillets, boneless
- 1 tablespoon lemon juice
- 3 teaspoons parsley, chopped
- Salt and pepper to the taste

Directions

1. In a bowl, mix the oil with the mustard and honey and whisk well.
2. Put the pecans and the parsley in another bowl.
3. Season the salmon fillets with salt and pepper, arrange them on a baking sheet lined with parchment paper, brush with the honey and mustard mix and top with the pecans mix.
4. Introduce in the oven at 400 degrees F, bake for 15 minutes, divide between plates, drizzle the lemon juice on top and serve.

Nutrition: calories 282; fat 15.5; fiber 8.5; carbs 20.9; protein 16.8

Shrimp And Mushrooms Mix

Servings: 4 | Cooking: 12 min

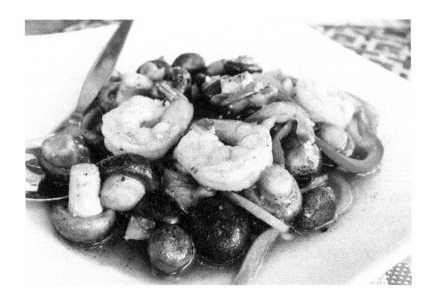

Ingredients

- 1 pound shrimp, peeled and deveined
- 2 green onions, sliced
- ½ pound white mushrooms, sliced
- 2 tablespoons balsamic vinegar
- 2 tablespoons sesame seeds, toasted
- 2 teaspoons ginger, minced
- 2 teaspoons garlic, minced
- 3 tablespoons olive oil

- 2 tablespoons dill, chopped

Directions

1. Heat up a pan with the oil over medium-high heat, add the green onions and the garlic and sauté for 2 minutes.
2. Add the rest of the ingredients except the shrimp and cook for 6 minutes more.
3. Add the shrimp, cook for 4 minutes, divide everything between plates and serve.

Nutrition: calories 245; fat 8.5; fiber 45.8; carbs 11.8; protein 17.7

Leeks And Calamari Mix

Servings: 6 | Cooking: 15 min

Ingredients

- 2 tablespoon avocado oil
- 2 leeks, chopped
- 1 red onion, chopped
- Salt and black to the taste
- 1 pound calamari rings
- 1 tablespoon parsley, chopped
- 1 tablespoon chives, chopped
- 2 tablespoons tomato paste

Directions

1. Heat up a pan with the avocado oil over medium heat, add the leeks and the onion, stir and sauté for 5 minutes.
2. Add the rest of the ingredients, toss, simmer over medium heat for 10 minutes, divide into bowls and serve.

Nutrition: calories 238; fat 9; fiber 5.6; carbs 14.4; protein 8.4

Cod With Lentils

Servings: 4 | Cooking: 30 min

Ingredients

- 1 red pepper, chopped
- 1 yellow onion, diced
- 1 teaspoon ground black pepper
- 1 teaspoon butter
- 1 jalapeno pepper, chopped
- ½ cup lentils
- 3 cups chicken stock
- 1 teaspoon salt
- 1 tablespoon tomato paste
- 1 teaspoon chili pepper
- 3 tablespoons fresh cilantro, chopped
- 8 oz cod, chopped

Directions

1. Place butter, red pepper, onion, and ground black pepper in the saucepan.
2. Roast the vegetables for 5 minutes over the medium heat.

3. Then add chopped jalapeno pepper, lentils, and chili pepper.
4. Mix up the mixture well and add chicken stock and tomato paste.
5. Stir until homogenous. Add cod.
6. Close the lid and cook chili for 20 minutes over the medium heat.

Nutrition: calories 187; fat 2.3; fiber 8.8; carbs 21.3; protein 20.6

Chapter 6: Salads & Side Dishes

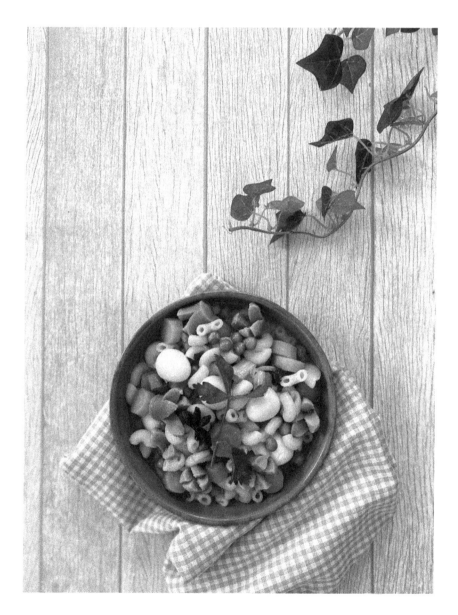

White Bean And Tuna Salad

Servings: 4 | Cooking: 8 min

Ingredients

- 1 (12 ounce) can solid white albacore tuna, drained
- 1 (16 ounce) can Great Northern beans, drained and rinsed
- 1 (2.25 ounce) can sliced black olives, drained
- 1 teaspoon dried oregano
- 1/2 teaspoon finely grated lemon zest
- 1/4 medium red onion, thinly sliced
- 3 tablespoons lemon juice
- 3/4-pound green beans, trimmed and snapped in half
- 4 large hard-cooked eggs, peeled and quartered
- 6 tablespoons extra-virgin olive oil
- Salt and ground black pepper, to taste

Directions

1. Place a saucepan on medium high fire. Add a cup of water and the green beans. Cover and cook for 8 minutes. Drain immediately once tender.

2. In a salad bowl, whisk well oregano, olive oil, lemon juice, and lemon zest. Season generously with pepper and salt and mix until salt is dissolved.
3. Stir in drained green beans, tuna, beans, olives, and red onion. Mix thoroughly to coat.
4. Adjust seasoning to taste.
5. Spread eggs on top.
6. Serve and enjoy.

Nutrition: Calories per serving: 551; Protein: 36.3g; Carbs: 33.4g; Fat: 30.3g

Beans And Spinach Mediterranean Salad

Servings: 4 | Cooking: 30 min

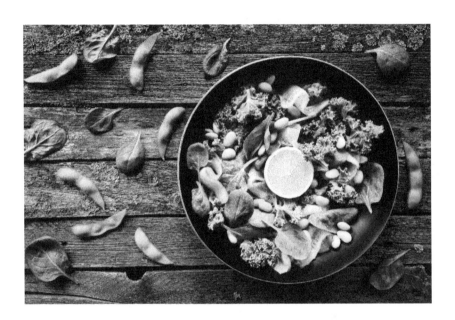

Ingredients

- 1 can (14 ounces) water-packed artichoke hearts, rinsed, drained and quartered
- 1 can (14-1/2 ounces) no-salt-added diced tomatoes, undrained
- 1 can (15 ounces) cannellini beans, rinsed and drained
- 1 small onion, chopped

- 1 tablespoon olive oil
- 1/4 teaspoon pepper
- 1/4 teaspoon salt
- 1/8 teaspoon crushed red pepper flakes
- 2 garlic cloves, minced
- 2 tablespoons Worcestershire sauce
- 6 ounces fresh baby spinach (about 8 cups)
- Additional olive oil, optional

Directions

1. Place a saucepan on medium high fire and heat for a minute.
2. Add oil and heat for 2 minutes. Stir in onion and sauté for 4 minutes. Add garlic and sauté for another minute.
3. Stir in seasonings, Worcestershire sauce, and tomatoes. Cook for 5 minutes while stirring continuously until sauce is reduced.
4. Stir in spinach, artichoke hearts, and beans. Sauté for 3 minutes until spinach is wilted and other ingredients are heated through.
5. Serve and enjoy.

Nutrition: Calories per serving: 187; Protein: 8.0g; Carbs: 30.0g; Fat: 4.0g

Grilled Veggie And Pasta With Marinara Sauce

Servings: 4 | Cooking: 30 min

Ingredients

- 8 oz whole wheat spaghetti
- 1 sweet onion, sliced into ¼-inch wide rounds
- 1 zucchini, sliced lengthwise
- 1 yellow summer squash, sliced lengthwise
- 2 red peppers, sliced into chunks
- 1/8 tsp freshly ground black pepper
- ½ tsp dried oregano
- 1 tsp sugar
- 1 tbsp chopped fresh basil or 1 tsp dried basil
- 2 tbsp chopped onion
- ½ tsp minced garlic
- salt
- 10 large fresh tomatoes, peeled and diced
- 2 tbsp extra virgin olive oil, divided

Directions

1. Make the marinara sauce by heating on medium high fire a tablespoon of oil in a large fry pan.

2. Sauté black pepper, oregano, sugar, basil, onions, garlic, salt and tomatoes. Once simmering, lower fire and allow to simmer for 30 minutes or until sauce has thickened.
3. Meanwhile, preheat broiler and grease baking pan with cooking spray.
4. Add sweet onion, zucchini, squash and red peppers in baking pan and brush with oil. Broil for 5 to 8 minutes or until vegetables are tender. Remove from oven and transfer veggies into a bowl.
5. Bring a large pot of water to a boil. Once boiling, add pasta and cook following manufacturer's instructions. Once al dente, drain and divide equally into 4 plates.
6. To serve, equally divide marinara sauce on to pasta, top with grilled veggies and enjoy.

Nutrition: Calories: Carbs: 41.9g; Protein: 8.3g; Fat: 6.2g

Chicken And Sweet Potato Stir Fry

Servings: 6 | Cooking: min

Ingredients

- ¼ tsp salt
- ½ cups quinoa, rinsed and drained
- 1 clove garlic, minced
- 1 cup frozen peas
- 1 cup water
- 1 jalapeno chili pepper, chopped
- 1 medium onion, chopped
- 1 medium-sized red bell pepper, chopped
- 1 tsp cumin, ground
- 1/8 tsp black pepper
- 12oz boneless chicken
- 1med sweet potatoes, cubed
- 3 tbsp fresh cilantro, chopped
- 4 tsp canola oil

Directions

1. Bring to a boil water and quinoa over medium heat. Simmer until the quinoa has absorbed the water.

2. In a small saucepan, put the sweet potatoes and enough water to cover the potatoes. Bring to a boil. Drain the potatoes and discard the water.

3. In a skillet, add the chicken and cook until brown. Transfer to a bowl.

4. Using the same skillet, heat 2 tablespoon of oil and sauté the onions and jalapeno pepper for one minute.

5. Add the bell pepper, cumin and garlic. Cook for three minutes until the vegetables have softened.

6. Add the peas and chicken. Cook for two minutes before adding the sweet potato and quinoa.

7. Stir cilantro and add salt and pepper to taste.

8. Serve and enjoy.

Nutrition: Calories: 187.6; Carbs: 18g; Protein: 16.3g; Fat: 5.6g

Shrimp Paella Made With Quinoa

Servings: 7 | Cooking: 40 min

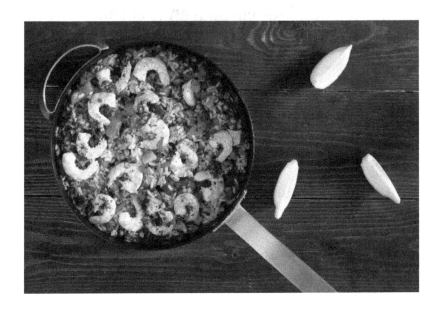

Ingredients

- 1 lb. large shrimp, peeled, deveined and thawed
- 1 tsp seafood seasoning
- 1 cup frozen green peas
- 1 red bell pepper, cored, seeded & membrane removed, sliced into ½" strips
- ½ cup sliced sun-dried tomatoes, packed in olive oil
- Salt to taste

- ½ tsp black pepper
- ½ tsp Spanish paprika
- ½ tsp saffron threads (optional turmeric)
- 1 bay leaf
- ¼ tsp crushed red pepper flakes
- 3 cups chicken broth; fat free, low sodium
- 1 ½ cups dry quinoa, rinse well
- 1 tbsp olive oil
- 2 cloves garlic, minced
- 1 yellow onion, diced

Directions

1. Season shrimps with seafood seasoning and a pinch of salt. Toss to mix well and refrigerate until ready to use.
2. Prepare and wash quinoa. Set aside.
3. On medium low fire, place a large nonstick skillet and heat oil. Add onions and for 5 minutes sauté until soft and tender.
4. Add paprika, saffron (or turmeric), bay leaves, red pepper flakes, chicken broth and quinoa. Season with salt and pepper.

5. Cover skillet and bring to a boil. Once boiling, lower fire to a simmer and cook until all liquid is absorbed, around ten minutes.
6. Add shrimp, peas and sun-dried tomatoes. For 5 minutes, cover and cook.
7. Once done, turn off fire and for ten minutes allow paella to set while still covered.
8. To serve, remove bay leaf and enjoy with a squeeze of lemon if desired.

Nutrition: Calories: 324.4; Protein: 22g; Carbs: 33g; Fat: 11.6g

Fasolakia – Potatoes & Green Beans In Olive Oil

Servings: 4 | Cooking: 25 min

Ingredients

- 1 1/2 onion, sliced thin
- 1 bunch of dill, chopped
- 1 cup water
- 1 large zucchini, quartered
- 1 lb. green beans frozen
- 1 tsp dried oregano
- 1/2 bunch parsley, chopped
- 1/2 cup extra virgin olive oil
- 15 oz can diced tomatoes
- 2 potatoes, quartered
- salt and pepper, to taste

Directions

1. Place a pot on medium high fire and heat pot for 2 minutes.
2. Add oil and heat for 3 minutes.

3. Stir in onions and sauté for 2 minutes. Stir in dill, oregano, and potatoes. Cook for 3 minutes. Season with pepper and salt.
4. Add dice tomatoes and water. Cover and simmer for 10 minutes.
5. Stir in zucchini and green beans. Cook for 5 minutes.
6. Adjust seasoning to taste, turn off fire, and stir in parsley.
7. Serve and enjoy.

Nutrition: Calories per serving: 384; Protein: 5.9g; Carbs: 30.6g; Fat: 27.9g

Pesto Pasta And Shrimps

Servings: 4 | Cooking: 15 min

Ingredients

- ¼ cup pesto, divided
- ¼ cup shaved Parmesan Cheese
- 1 ¼ lbs. large shrimp, peeled and deveined
- 1 cup halved grape tomatoes
- 4-oz angel hair pasta, cooked, rinsed and drained

Directions

1. On medium high fire, place a nonstick large fry pan and grease with cooking spray.
2. Add tomatoes, pesto and shrimp. Cook for 15 minutes or until shrimps are opaque, while covered.
3. Stir in cooked pasta and cook until heated through.
4. Transfer to a serving plate and garnish with Parmesan cheese.

Nutrition: Calories: 319; Carbs: 23.6g; Protein: 31.4g; Fat: 11g

Seafood And Veggie Pasta

Servings: 4 | Cooking: 20 min

Ingredients

- ¼ tsp pepper
- ¼ tsp salt
- 1 lb raw shelled shrimp
- 1 lemon, cut into wedges
- 1 tbsp butter
- 1 tbsp olive oil
- 2 5-oz cans chopped clams, drained (reserve 2 tbsp clam juice)
- 2 tbsp dry white wine
- 4 cloves garlic, minced
- 4 cups zucchini, spiraled (use a veggie spiralizer)
- 4 tbsp Parmesan Cheese
- Chopped fresh parsley to garnish

Directions

1. Ready the zucchini and spiralize with a veggie spiralizer. Arrange 1 cup of zucchini noodle per bowl. Total of 4 bowls.

2. On medium fire, place a large nonstick saucepan and heat oil and butter.
3. For a minute, sauté garlic. Add shrimp and cook for 3 minutes until opaque or cooked.
4. Add white wine, reserved clam juice and clams. Bring to a simmer and continue simmering for 2 minutes or until half of liquid has evaporated. Stir constantly.
5. Season with pepper and salt. And if needed add more to taste.
6. Remove from fire and evenly distribute seafood sauce to 4 bowls.
7. Top with a tablespoonful of Parmesan cheese per bowl, serve and enjoy.

Nutrition: Calories: 324.9; Carbs: 12g; Protein: 43.8g; Fat: 11.3g

Cilantro-dijon Vinaigrette On Kidney Bean Salad

Servings: 4 | Cooking: 0 min

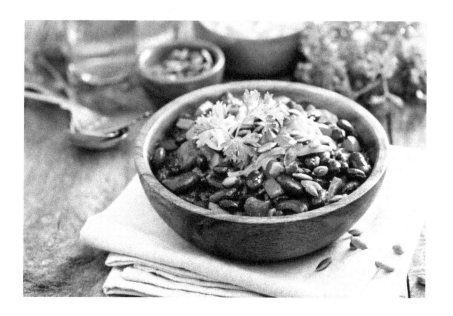

Ingredients

- 1 15-oz. can kidney beans, drained and rinsed
- 1/2 English cucumbers, chopped
- 1 Medium-sized heirloom tomato, chopped
- 1 bunch fresh cilantro, stems removed, chopped (about 1 1/4 cup)
- 1 red onion, chopped (about 1 cup)
- 1 large lime or lemon, juice of

- 3 tbsp Private Reserve or Early Harvest Greek extra virgin olive oil
- 1 tsp Dijon mustard
- ½ tsp fresh garlic paste, or finely chopped garlic
- 1 tsp sumac
- Salt and pepper, to taste

Directions

1. In a small bowl, whisk well all vinaigrette ingredients.
2. In a salad bowl, combine cilantro chopped veggies, and kidney beans.
3. Add vinaigrette to salad and toss well to mix.
4. For 30 minutes allow for flavors to mix and set in the fridge.
5. Mix and adjust seasoning if needed before serving.

Nutrition: Calories per serving: 154; Protein: 5.5g; Carbs: 18.3g; Fat: 7.4g

Tasty Mushroom Bolognese

Servings: 6 | Cooking: 65 min

Ingredients

- ¼ cup chopped fresh parsley
- 1.5 oz Parmigiano-Reggiano cheese, grated
- 1 tbsp kosher salt
- 10-oz whole wheat spaghetti, cooked and drained
- ¼ cup milk
- 1 14-oz can whole peeled tomatoes
- ½ cup white wine
- 2 tbsp tomato paste
- 1 tbsp minced garlic
- 8 cups finely chopped cremini mushrooms
- ½ lb. ground pork
- ½ tsp freshly ground black pepper, divided
- ¾ tsp kosher salt, divided
- 2 ½ cups chopped onion
- 1 tbsp olive oil
- 1 cup boiling water
- ½-oz dried porcini mushrooms

Directions

1. Let porcini stand in a boiling bowl of water for twenty minutes, drain (reserve liquid), rinse and chop. Set aside.
2. On medium high fire, place a Dutch oven with olive oil and cook for ten minutes cook pork, ¼ tsp pepper, ¼ tsp salt and onions. Constantly mix to break ground pork pieces.
3. Stir in ¼ tsp pepper, ¼ tsp salt, garlic and cremini mushrooms. Continue cooking until liquid has evaporated, around fifteen minutes.
4. Stirring constantly, add porcini and sauté for a minute.
5. Stir in wine, porcini liquid, tomatoes and tomato paste. Let it simmer for forty minutes. Stir occasionally. Pour milk and cook for another two minutes before removing from fire.
6. Stir in pasta and transfer to a serving dish. Garnish with parsley and cheese before serving.

Nutrition: Calories: 358; Carbs: 32.8g; Protein: 21.1g; Fat: 15.4g

Chapter 7: Dessert Recipes

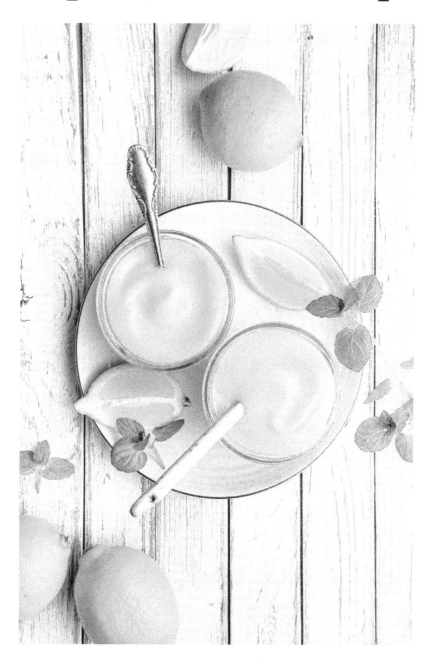

Lime Vanilla Fudge

Servings: 6 | Cooking: 0 min

Ingredients

- 1/3 cup cashew butter
- 5 tablespoons lime juice
- ½ teaspoon lime zest, grated
- 1 tablespoons stevia

Directions

1. In a bowl, mix the cashew butter with the other ingredients and whisk well.
2. Line a muffin tray with parchment paper, scoop 1 tablespoon of lime fudge mix in each of the muffin tins and keep in the freezer for 3 hours before serving.

Nutrition: calories 200; fat 4.5; fiber 3.4; carbs 13.5; protein 5

Pear Sauce

Servings: 6 | Cooking: 15 min

Ingredients

- 10 pears, sliced
- 1 cup apple juice
- 1 1/2 tsp cinnamon
- 1/4 tsp nutmeg

Directions

1. Add all ingredients into the instant pot and stir well.
2. Seal pot with lid and cook on high for 15 minutes.
3. Once done, allow to release pressure naturally for 10 minutes then release remaining using quick release. Remove lid.
4. Blend the pear mixture using an immersion blender until smooth.
5. Serve and enjoy.

Nutrition: Calories 222 Fat 0.6 g Carbohydrates 58.2 g Sugar 38 g Protein 1.3 g Cholesterol 0 mg

Honey Cream

Servings: 2 | Cooking: 5 min

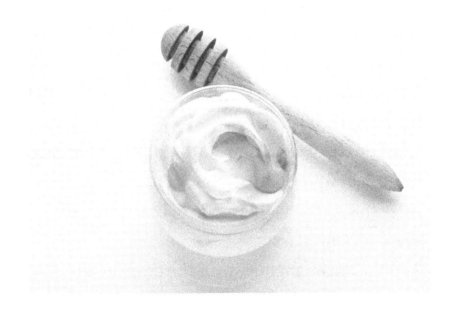

Ingredients

- ½ cup cream
- ¼ cup milk
- 2 teaspoons honey
- 1 teaspoon vanilla extract
- 1 tablespoons gelatin
- 2 tablespoons orange juice

Directions

1. Mix up together milk and gelatin and leave it for 5 minutes.
2. Meanwhile, pour cream in the saucepan and bring it to boil.
3. Add honey and vanilla extract.
4. Remove the cream from the heat and stir well until honey is dissolved.
5. After this, add gelatin mixture (milk+gelatin) and mix it up until gelatin is dissolved.
6. After this, place 1 tablespoon of orange juice in every serving glass.
7. Add the cream mixture over the orange juice.
8. Refrigerate the pannacotta for 30-50 minutes in the fridge or until it is solid.

Nutrition: calories 100; fat 4; fiber 0; carbs 11; protein 4.6

Dragon Fruit, Pear, And Spinach Salad

Servings: 4 | Cooking: 3 min

Ingredients

- 5 ounces spinach leaves, torn
- 1 dragon fruit, peeled then cubed
- 2 pears, peeled then cubed
- 10 ounces organic goat cheese
- 1 cup pecan, halves
- 6 ounces blackberries
- 6 ounces raspberries
- 8 tablespoons olive oil
- 8 tablespoons red wine vinegar
- 1 tablespoon poppy seeds

Directions

1. In a mixing bowl, combine all Ingredients: except for the poppy seeds.
2. Place inside the fridge and allow to chill before serving.
3. Sprinkle with poppy seeds on top before serving.

Nutrition: Calories per serving:321; Carbs: 27.2g; Protein: 3.3g; Fat: 3.1g

Mediterranean Biscotti

Servings: 3 | Cooking: 1 Hour

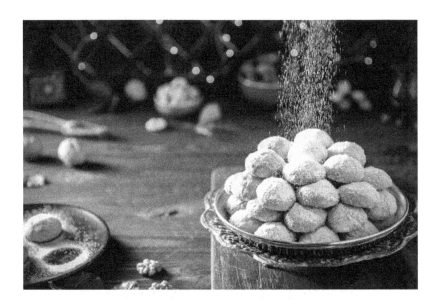

Ingredients

- 2 eggs
- 1 cups whole-wheat flour
- 1 cup all-purpose flour
- 3/4 cup parmesan cheese, grated
- 2 teaspoons baking powder
- 2 tablespoons sugar
- 1/4 cup sun-dried tomato, finely chopped
- 1/4 cup Kalamata olive, finely chopped

- 1/3 cup olive oil
- 1/2 teaspoon salt
- 1/2 teaspoon black pepper, cracked
- 1 teaspoon dried oregano (preferably Greek)
- 1 teaspoon dried basil

Directions

1. Into a large-sized bowl, beat the eggs and the sugar together. Pour in the olive; beat until smooth.
2. In another bowl, combine the flours, baking powder, pepper, salt, oregano, and basil. Stir the flour mix into the egg mixture, stirring until blended.
3. Stir in the cheese, tomatoes, and olives; stirring until thoroughly combined.
4. Divide the dough into 2 portions; shape each into 10-inch long logs. Place the logs into a parchment-lined cookie sheet; flatten the log tops slightly.
5. Bake for about 30 minutes in a preheated 375F oven or until the logs are pale golden and not quite firm to the touch.

6. Remove from the oven; let cool on the baking sheet for 3 minutes. Transfer the logs into a cutting board; slice each log into 1/2-inch diagonal slices using a serrated knife.

7. Place the biscotti slices on the baking sheet, return into the 325F oven, and bake for about 20 to 25 minutes until dry and firm. Flip the slices halfway through baking. Remove from the oven, transfer on a wire rack and let cool.

Nutrition:731.6 Cal, 36.5 g total fat (9 g sat. fat), 146 mg chol., 1238.4 mg sodium, 77.8 g carb., 3.5 g fiber, 10.7 g sugar, and 23.3 g protein.

Kataifi

Servings: 8-10 | Cooking: 30 min

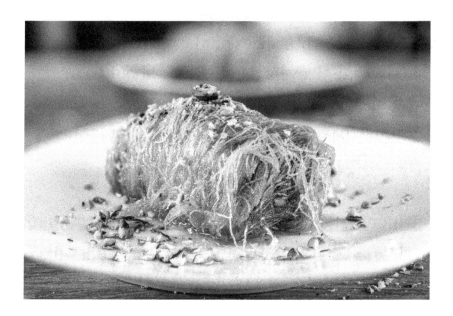

Ingredients

- 1 kilogram almonds, blanched and then chopped
- 1 teaspoon cinnamon
- 1/4 kilogram kataifi phyllo
- 2 eggs
- 4 tablespoons sugar
- 400 g butter
- 1 1/2 kilograms sugar
- 1 lemon rind

- 1 teaspoon lemon juice
- 5 cups water

Directions

1. Preheat the oven to 170C.
2. Put the sugar, eggs, cinnamon, and the almonds in a bowl.
3. With your fingers, open the kataifi pastry gently. Lay it on a piece of marble and wood. Put 1 tablespoon of the almond mixture in one end and then roll the pastry into a log or a cylinder. Make sure you fold the pastry a little tight so the filling is enclosed securely. Repeat the process with the remaining pastry and almond mixture.
4. Melt the butter and put into a baking dish.
5. Brush the kataifi rolls with the melted butter, covering all the sides.
6. Place into baking sheets and bake for about 30 minutes.
7. Meanwhile, prepare the syrup.
8. Except for the lemon juice, cook the rest of the syrup ingredients for about 5-10 minutes. Add the lemon juice and let cook for a few minutes until the syrup is slightly thick.

9. After baking the kataifi, pour the syrup over the still warm rolls.

10. Cover the pastry with a clean towel. Let cool as the kataifi absorbs the syrup.

Nutrition:1085 cal., 83.3 total fat (24.6 g sat. fat), 119 mg chol., 248 mg sodium, 759 mg pot., 76.6 g total carbs., 12.7 g fiber, 59.1 g sugar, and 22.6 g protein.

Walnuts Kataifi

Servings: 2 | Cooking: 50 min

Ingredients

- 7 oz kataifi dough
- 1/3 cup walnuts, chopped
- ½ teaspoon ground cinnamon
- ¾ teaspoon vanilla extract
- 4 tablespoons butter, melted
- ¼ teaspoon ground clove
- 1/3 cup water
- 3 tablespoons honey

Directions

1. For the filling: mix up together walnuts, ground cinnamon, and vanilla extract. Add ground clove and blend the mixture until smooth.
2. Make the kataifi dough: grease the casserole mold with butter and place ½ part of kataifi dough.
3. Then sprinkle the filling over the kataifi dough.
4. After this, sprinkle the filling with 1 tablespoon of melted butter.
5. Sprinkle the filling with remaining kataifi dough.

6. Make the roll from ½ part of kataifi dough and cut it.
7. Gently arrange the kataifi roll in the tray.
8. Repeat the same steps with remaining dough. In the end, you should get 2 kataifi rolls.
9. Preheat the oven to 355F and place the tray with kataifi rolls inside.
10. Bake the dessert for 50 minutes or until it is crispy.
11. Meanwhile, make the syrup: bring the water to boil.
12. Add honey and heat it up until the honey is dissolved.
13. When the kataifi rolls are cooked, pour the hot syrup over the hot kataifi rolls.
14. Cut every kataifi roll on 2 pieces.
15. Serve the dessert with remaining syrup.

Nutrition: calories 120; fat 1.5; fiber 0; carbs 22; protein 3

Cinnamon Tea

Servings: 1 Cup | Cooking: 32 min

Ingredients

- 6 cups water
- 1 (3-in.) cinnamon stick
- 6 TB. Ahmad Tea, Ceylon tea, or your favorite
- 3 TB. Sugar

Directions

1. In a teapot over low heat, bring water and cinnamon stick to a simmer for 30 minutes. Remove cinnamon stick.
2. Stir in Ahmad tea and sugar, and simmer for 2 minutes.
3. Remove from heat, and let sit for 10 minutes.
4. Strain tea into tea cups, and serve warm.

Tiny Orange Cardamom Cookies

Servings: 80 | Cooking: 12 min

Ingredients

- 1/2 cup whole-wheat flour
- 1/2 cup all-purpose flour
- 1 large egg
- 1 tablespoon sesame seeds, toasted, optional (salted roasted pistachios, chopped)
- 1 teaspoon orange zest
- 1 teaspoon vanilla extract
- 1/2 cup butter, softened
- 1/2 cup sugar
- 1/4 teaspoon ground cardamom

Directions

1. Preheat the oven to 375F.
2. In a medium bowl, blend the orange zest and the sugar thoroughly, and then blend in the cardamom.
3. Add the butter and with a mixer, beat until the mixture is fluffy and light. Beat in the egg and the vanilla into the mixture.

4. With the mixer on low speed, mix in the flours into the mixture.
5. Line 3 baking sheets with parchment paper. Using a level teaspoon measure, drop batter of the cookie mixture onto the sheets.
6. Top each cookie with a pinch of sesame seeds or nuts, if desired; bake for 1bout 10-12 minutes or until the cookies are brown at the edges and crisp.
7. When baked, transfer the cookies on a cooling rack and let them cool completely.

Nutrition:113 Cal, 1.4 g protein, 6.5 g total fat (3.8 g sat. fat) 12 g total carbs., 0.3 g fiber, 46 mg sodium, and 29 mg chol.

Chocolate Ganache

Preparation: 10 min | Cooking: 3 min | Servings: 16

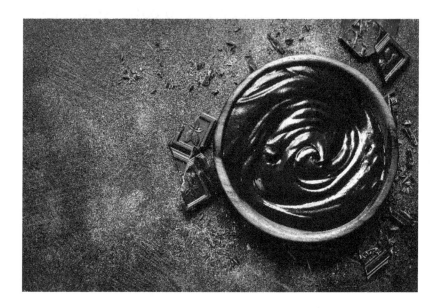

Ingredients

- 9 ounces bittersweet chocolate, chopped
- cup heavy cream
- 1 tablespoon dark rum (optional)

Directions

1. Put the chocolate in a medium bowl. Heat the cream in a small saucepan over medium heat.

2. Bring to a boil. When the cream has reached a boiling point, pour the chopped chocolate over it and beat until smooth. Stir the rum if desired.
3. Allow the ganache to cool slightly before you pour it on a cake. Begin in the middle of the cake and work outside. For a fluffy icing or chocolate filling, let it cool until thick and beat with a whisk until light and fluffy.

Nutrition: 142 calories; 10.8g fat; 1.4g protein

CPSIA information can be obtained
at www.ICGtesting.com
Printed in the USA
BVHW092303210621
610124BV00010B/2337